Fabulous Faux-Fisl

Plant-Based Seafood Recipes

BY

Christina Tosch

Copyright Notes

Table of Contents

Introduction

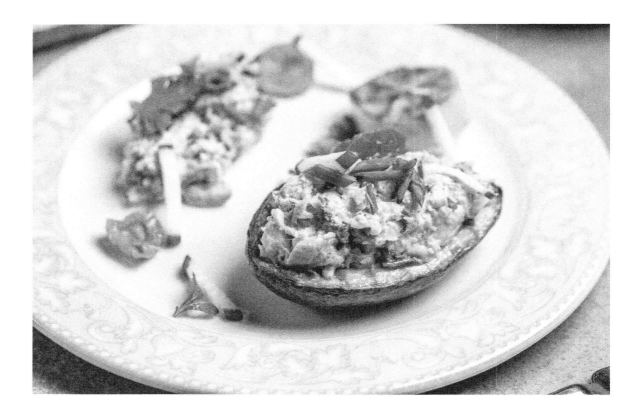

There are so many reasons not to eat meat, and the same goes for seafood. Fish are way more intelligent than you think, they do feel pain, and are often caught via painful and sometimes horrific means. What's more, current fishing rates mean that our ocean ecosystems are in danger of collapse by 2050.

There are lots of mock meat products on the store shelves, but that's not always the case when it comes to sourcing faux-fish and plant-based seafood. The reason for this is because fish has a unique texture and flavor that makes it difficult to imitate.

These 40 fabulous faux-fish and plant-based seafood recipes will show you how King Oyster mushrooms can replace lobster, how to use seafood flakes to add a salty flavor and replicate meaty pan-seared tuna using watermelon.

Better yet, all of these plant-based seafoods and faux-fish recipes can be easily adapted for anyone following a vegan-friendly diet.

As anyone who enjoys plant-based seafood will tell you, there is no need to sacrifice our oceans in the quest for amazing food.

Artichoke 'Lobster' Rolls

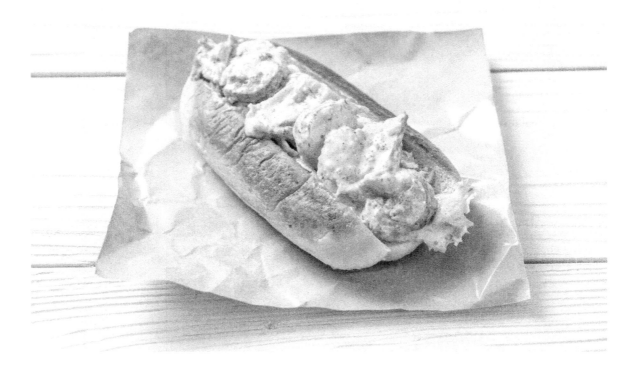

Seaweed flakes and Old Bay seasoning will add a real taste of the sea to these artichoke lobster-free rolls.

Servings: 4-6

Total Time: 15mins

Ingredients:

- 1 tbsp olive oil
- 2 (12 ounce) jars of artichoke hearts (rinsed)
- ¼ tsp dulse powder
- ¼ tsp Old Bay seasoning
- 2 garlic cloves (peeled and minced)
- 2 celery ribs (minced)
- 2 tbsp parsley (minced)
- 1 tbsp freshly squeezed lemon juice
- Sea salt and ground black pepper
- ¼-½ cup mayonnaise
- Soft hot dog buns (split, toasted, and buttered)

Directions:

1. Over moderate heat, heat the oil in a skillet.

2. Add the artichokes to the skillet along with the dulse and Old Bay seasoning. Cook, while stirring for 6-8 minutes, or until lightly charred and browned.

3. Add the garlic and cook for an additional 2-3 minutes. Remove and transfer to a bowl to slightly cool.

4. To the bowl, add the celery, parsley, fresh lemon juice, salt, black pepper, and mayonnaise. Combine gently, taste, and season.

5. Toast and butter the soft dog buns. Fill with the artichoke mixture and enjoy.

Asparagus and Lobster Mushroom Risotto

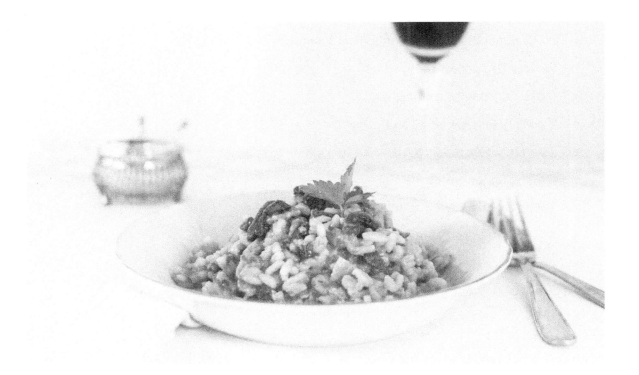

If a dish calls for lobster, why not switch to cruelty-free lobster mushrooms? They have a great seafood-like flavor, vibrant color, and pair exceptionally well with rice dishes.

Servings: 4

Total Time: 1hour

Ingredients:

- 1 pound fresh asparagus
- Drizzle of olive oil (as needed)
- 1 cup lobster mushrooms (coarsely chopped)
- 4 tbsp butter (divided)
- 1 cup Arborio rice
- 2-3 cups vegetable stock
- ½ cup Parmesan cheese (freshly and finely grated)
- Sea salt (to season)

Directions:

1. Snap the bottoms of the asparagus stalks to find out where the stalk if most tender. Cut the remaining stalks where the asparagus snaps.

2. Arrange on a baking tray and drizzle all over with oil.

3. Bake the asparagus in the oven at 400 degrees F until tender; this will take 15-18 minutes. Remove from the oven and coarsely chop.

4. Add the chopped mushrooms to a small frying pan along with 1 tablespoon of butter. Sauté until soft and tender for around 15-20 minutes.

5. Heat 2 tablespoons of butter in a pan.

6. Add the rice to the pan and over moderate heat, stir to toast.

7. One cup at a time, pour in the stock, while frequently stirring until the rice has absorbed the liquid.

8. After around 15-20 minutes, and when the rice is tender, add the remaining butter along with the cheese.

9. Fold in the roasted asparagus and top with the sautéed mushrooms.

10. Season the risotto with salt and enjoy.

Baked Shiitake Mushroom "Shrimp"

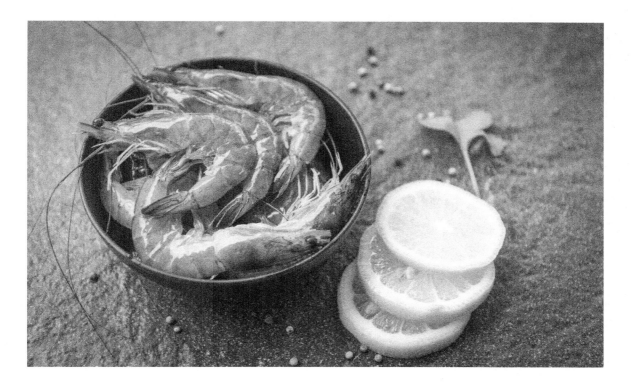

These mushrooms offer just the same perfect amount of crisp and crunch as fried shrimp. Serve on a bed of lettuce, with a cocktail sauce dip or both!

Servings: 20

Total Time: 35mins

Ingredients:

Beer Batter:

- ½ cup flour (of choice, gluten-free)
- ¼ cup beer (of choice, gluten-free)

Breading:

- ¾ cup panko breadcrumbs
- ¼ tsp dried basil
- ¼ tsp dried thyme
- ¼ tsp dried oregano
- ¼ tsp salt
- 1 tbsp olive oil

Shrimp:

- 10 medium shitake mushroom tops (sliced in half)
- Sea salt (to season)
- Fresh lemon wedges (to serve)

Directions:

1. Preheat the main oven to 425 degrees F. Using parchment paper, line a baking sheet.

2. First, prepare the batter. In a shallow dish or bowl, combine the flour with the beer, whisking to form a pancake batter-like consistency. Add more flour or beer as needed.

3. In a second dish or bowl, combine the breadcrumbs with the basil, thyme, oregano, salt, and oil. Stir the mixture well to create a sand-like consistency.

4. Dip the sliced mushrooms first in the batter and second in the breading, making sure they are evenly and well coated. The easiest way to achieve this is to pick up and dip the mushroom using a fork.

5. Arrange the mushrooms on a baking sheet and bake in the preheated oven for 7-10 minutes. Flip the mushrooms over and bake on the other side for 7-10 minutes, until they are golden all over.

6. Remove from the oven and season with sea salt.

7. Serve with a squeeze of lemon juice and enjoy.

Baked Tuna-Free Casserole

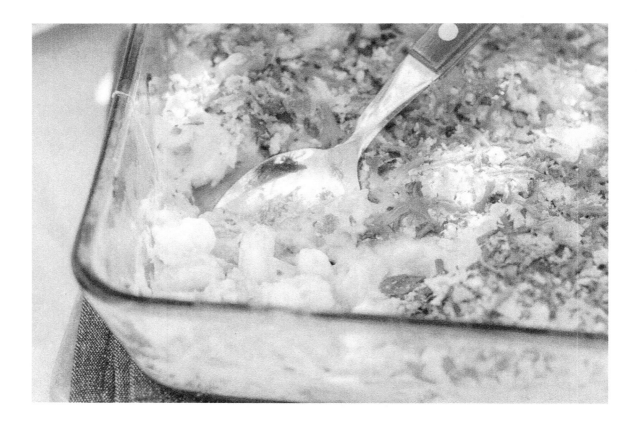

An oven-baked casserole is the ultimate fuss-free, family-friendly meal. Enjoy this delicious tuna-style casserole safe in the knowledge you aren't putting further pressure on the fishing industry and the ocean life it exploits.

Servings: 4

Total Time: 1hour 15mins

Ingredients:

Sauce:

- 2½ cups soy milk
- 1 tsp onion powder
- ½ cup unsalted cashews
- ½ tsp black pepper
- 1 tbsp kelp powder

Casserole:

- 1½ cups uncooked elbow pasta
- 1 yellow onion (peeled and diced)
- 8 white mushrooms (sliced)
- 2 cups frozen green peas
- 2 (15 ounce) cans garbanzo beans (drained)

Directions:

1. Preheat the main oven to 375 degrees F.

2. First, make the sauce. Add the soy milk, onion powder, cashews, black pepper, and kelp powder to a food processor and blitz until smooth. Transfer to a bowl and set to one side.

3. Cook the elbow pasta using packet instructions. Drain away the water leaving the pasta in the cooking pot. Take off the heat.

4. Place a skillet over high heat. Add the onions and mushrooms and sauté for 3-4 minutes until softened. Add the onions and mushrooms to the pasta along with the frozen peas.

5. Add the garbanzo beans to the food processor and pulse until chunky but not pureed. Transfer to the pasta pot.

6. Pour the set-aside sauce into the pot. Stir the whole mixture to combine then transfer to a 9x13" casserole dish.

7. Place in the oven and bake for 35-40 until golden brown.

8. Take out of the oven and allow to cool for 5 minutes before serving.

Banana Blossom Faux "Fish"

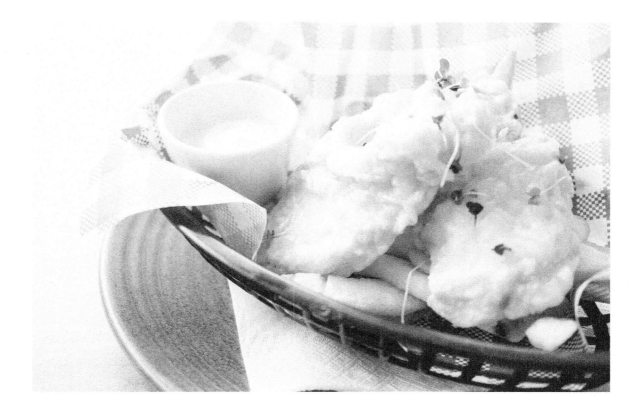

Are you following a plant-based diet but missing the flavor of fish? Then this recipe is the one for you. The secret to success lies in the garnishes and side dishes. So, serve with tartar sauce, and garnish with dill and a squeeze of lemon. All three will help to provide a fabulous fish flavor.

Servings: 8

Total Time: 20mins

Ingredients:

Flour Mixture:

- 1 cup all-purpose flour
- ½ tsp salt
- 1 tsp dill
- 1½ tbsp nori (crushed)

Batter:

- 1 cup flour
- ½ tsp salt
- Pinch of turmeric
- 2 tbsp pickle juice
- 2 tsp freshly squeezed lemon juice
- ½ cup sparkling water

Fish;

- Oil (to fry)
- 1 (20 ounce) canned banana blossoms in brine (rinsed and brined)
- Tartare sauce, store-bought (to serve)
- Fresh dill (to garnish)
- Lemon wedges (to squeeze)

Directions:

1. In separate shallow bowls, combine the all-purpose flour, salt dill, and crushed nori.

2. In the second bowl, whisk the flour, salt, turmeric, pickle juice, fresh lemon juice, and sparkling water to incorporate.

3. In a wok or pot, heat the oil for frying. The banana blossoms should swim in the frying oil but take care not to overfill the pot.

4. Coat the blossoms in the flour-sparkling water mixture. Next, dip them in the batter.

5. Lower the coated blossoms carefully into the oil and fry for 4-5 minutes, or until golden. You will need to flip them over once to ensure an even fry.

6. Transfer the golden blossoms to a kitchen paper towel line plate.

7. Serve with tartar sauce, garnish with fresh dill and a squeeze of lemon juice.

Beer Battered Faux-Fish Tacos with Mango Salsa

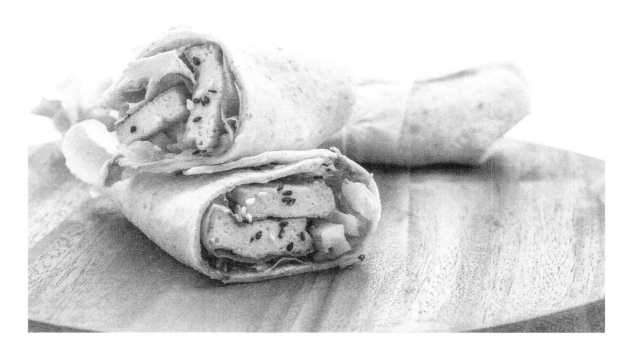

Fake it and make it! Ditch the take-out and instead opt for beer-battered seafood-free tacos with fruity homemade mango salsa.

Servings: 8

Total Time: 30mins

Ingredients

Tofu:

- 3 (14 ounce) packages of extra firm tofu (not silken)
- 1 cup beer
- 1 cup all-purpose flour
- 1 cup panko breadcrumbs
- 1½ tsp finely ground sea salt
- 1 tbsp Old Bay seasoning
- 1-2 cups canola oil

Salsa:

- 2 fresh corn cobs
- 2 mangoes (pitted, and finely diced)
- 1 small red onion (peeled and finely diced)
- 1 jalapeno pepper (seeded and finely chopped)
- ½ cup cilantro leaves (coarsely chopped)
- 20 cherry tomatoes (finely diced)
- Freshly squeezed juice from 1 large lime
- Finely ground sea salt (to season)
- 8 corn tortillas

Directions:

1. Press the tofu between 2 plates lined with kitchen paper towels, for 20-25 minutes. Slice the pressed tofu into ½ "thick, 3" long, and 1" wide pieces.

2. To prepare the salsa: Grill the corn, on the cob, until grill marks appear all over, for approximately 15-20 minutes. Slice the kernels off the cob.

3. Add the mango to a bowl along with the onion, grilled corn kernels, jalapeno, cilantro, tomatoes, fresh lime juice, and salt. Stir the mixture well to combine.

4. For the faux-fish, add the beer to one shallow bowl, the flour to a second shallow bowl, and the panko to a third shallow bowl.

5. Whisk the salt and Old Bay seasoning into the flour until incorporated.

6. Dip the tofu first in the flour, then second in the beer, and finally dredge through the panko until evenly and thoroughly coated all over. Transfer to a plate until you are ready to fry.

7. Line a cookie sheet with kitchen paper towels.

8. Add canola oil to a deep skillet to around 1" deep, and on moderately high heat, heat the oil.

9. Once hope, add each tofu pieces to the pan and fry for 3-5 minutes, until golden. You will need to use kitchen tongs to flip the tofu over before frying until golden for another 3-5 minutes.

10. Transfer the fried tofu to the kitchen paper towel-lined cookie sheet.

11. Fill the corn tortillas with 2-3 pieces of fried tofu and top with the homemade salsa.

Carrot Lox

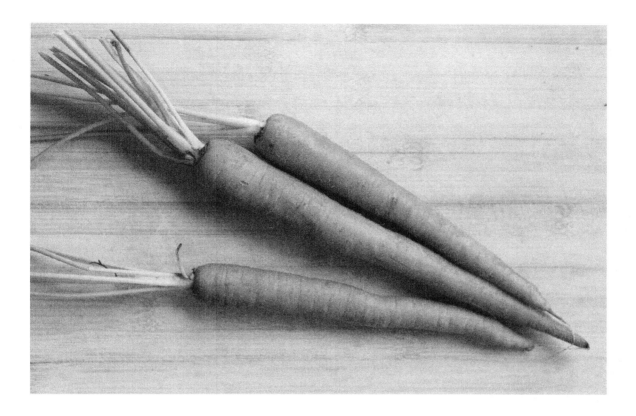

Equally as colorful and flavorful as smoked salmon, this carrot lox makes the ideal brunch or lunch treat.

Servings: 4

Total Time: 5mins

Ingredients:

- 14 ounces large carrots (peeled into thin ribbons)
- 1 tsp liquid smoke
- 2 tsp tamari sauce
- 1 tbsp rice vinegar
- 2 tbsp sunflower oil
- 1 tbsp flax oil
- ¼-½ tsp sea salt
- 1 tsp maple syrup
- 1 nori sheet (cut into pieces)
- Toasted bagels (to serve, optional)
- Vegan cream cheese (to serve, optional)
- Freshly squeezed lemon juice (to serve, optional)

Directions:

1. Steam the carrot ribbons for approximately 5 minutes, until soft but not mushy.

2. Remove the carrots from the steamer and transfer to a bowl to slightly cool.

3. Prepare a marinade. In a second bowl, combine the liquid smoke with the tamari sauce, rice vinegar, sunflower oil, flax oil, sea salt, and maple syrup.

4. Add the warm carrots to the marinade and toss gently to coat.

5. Transfer to an airtight container. Add the nori sheet to the container and seal.

6. Place in the fridge overnight.

7. Serve with toasted bagels, vegan cheese, and a squeeze of fresh lemon juice.

Garbanzo Bean "Tuna" Toast

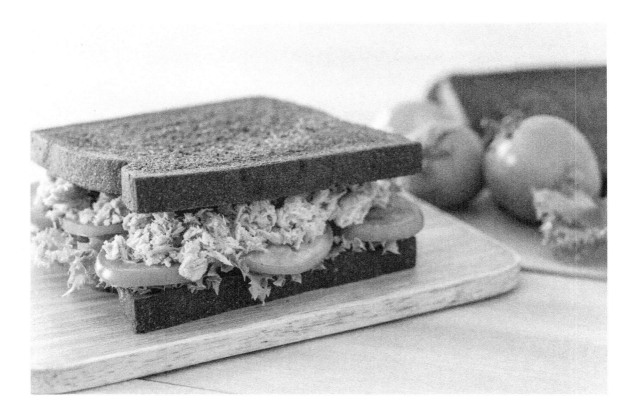

Say 'so long' to seafood and instead opt for this garbanzo bean toast instead of the regular tuna topping.

Servings: 3

Total Time: 15mins

Ingredients:

- ¼ cup sunflower seeds
- 1 (15 ounce) can garbanzo beans (drained and rinsed)
- 1 small red bell pepper (cored and diced)
- 3 green onions (finely chopped)
- 2 tbsp mayonnaise
- 1 tsp Dijon mustard
- Freshly squeezed juice of 1 lemon
- ¼ tsp garlic powder
- Pinch of sea salt and black pepper
- 6 slices rye bread (toasted)

Directions:

1. In a pan, cook the sunflower seeds over moderate to low heat until golden brown, for 4-6 minutes. You need to shake the pan a few times while they cook to ensure an even toast. Put to one side to cool.

2. To a food processor, add the garbanzo beans and toasted sunflower seed and process on pulse until finely chopped.

3. Transfer the mixture from the processor to a bowl and add the bell pepper along with the green onion.

4. Stir in the mayonnaise, mustard, fresh lemon juice, and garlic powder. Season the mayo mixture to taste, with salt and black pepper and mix until combined.

5. Spread the mixture on top of the rye toast and serve straight away.

Citrus Avocado Ceviche

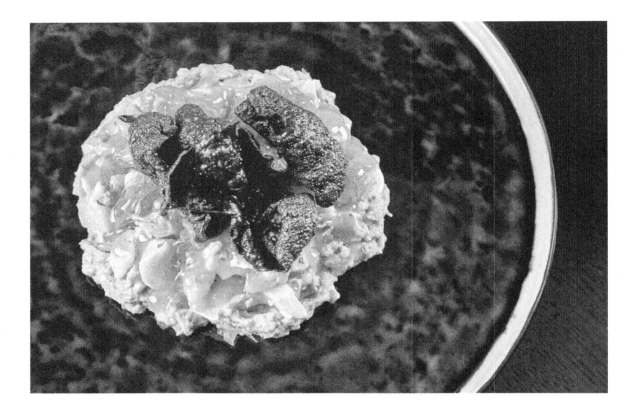

Ceviche is a Peruvian dish that uses citrus juice to "cook" raw seafood. To enjoy this South American classic, swap fish for creamy avocado and juicy fruit and serve with crisp tortilla chips.

Servings: 6

Total Time: 15mins

Ingredients:

- 1 large ruby red grapefruit (peeled, sliced into rounds)
- 2 oranges (peeled, sliced into rounds)
- 2 ripe avocadoes (peeled, destoned, diced)
- ½ cup red onion (diced)
- ½ jalapeno (deseeded, diced)
- ½ cup fresh cilantro (chopped)
- Juice of 2 limes
- ½ tsp sea salt
- Tortilla chips (to serve)

Directions:

1. Gently tug the grapefruit and orange rounds apart and separate them into small triangles and transfer to a large bowl.

2. Add the avocado, red onion, jalapeno, cilantro, lime juice, and sea salt to the bowl. Toss gently to combine.

3. Serve the ceviche straight away with tortilla chips for dipping.

Coconut-Crusted Faux-Fish Sticks with Dill Mayonnaise

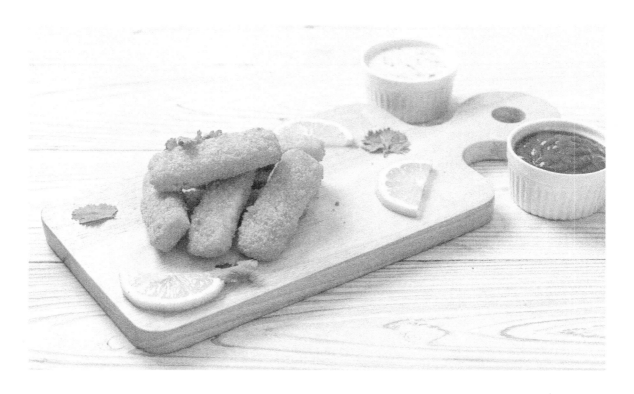

Hearts of Palm have great texture and are an ideal replacement for seafood. Serve with a creamy homemade dill mayonnaise dip.

Servings: N/A*

Total Time: 35mins

Ingredients:

Fingers:

- 1 (14 ounce) can of hearts of palm (drained)
- ½ tsp sea salt
- ½ tsp garlic powder
- ½ cup + 2 tbsp brown rice flour
- ½ cup dairy-free milk
- ¼ cup cornflour
- ½ cup desiccated coconut

Dill Mayonnaise:

- ¼ cup mayonnaise
- 2 tbsp fresh dill (chopped)
- 1 tbsp capers

Directions:

1. Preheat the main oven to 375 degrees F. Using parchment paper line, a baking tray.

2. Transfer the drained hearts of palm to a bowl.

3. Using two metal forks, tear and rip the hearts of palm into thin, stringy pieces. Make sure that no long size or chunky pieces remain.

4. Season with sea salt, garlic powder, and 2 tablespoons brown rice flour.

5. Add the remaining brown rice flour to a shallow bowl.

6. In a second bowl, add the milk and whisk in the cornflour.

7. In another bowl, add the desiccated coconut.

8. One at a time, take one heaped tablespoon of the hearts of palm and roll into a sausage shape. Flatter the sausage into a fish stick-like shape.

9. Coat the fish stick in the brown rice flour, and then dip into the milk mixture, and finally the desiccated coconut. Repeat the process until all of the mixtures is used.

10. Transfer the fish sticks onto the parchment-lined baking tray.

11. Transfer to the oven for 25-30 minutes, until golden.

12. For the dill mayonnaise: In a bowl, whisk the mayonnaise with the fresh dill and capers. Keep chilled until ready to serve.

13. Serve the fish sticks with the dill mayonnaise on the side.

*The number of sticks will depend on their size

Cod-Free Baccala Salad

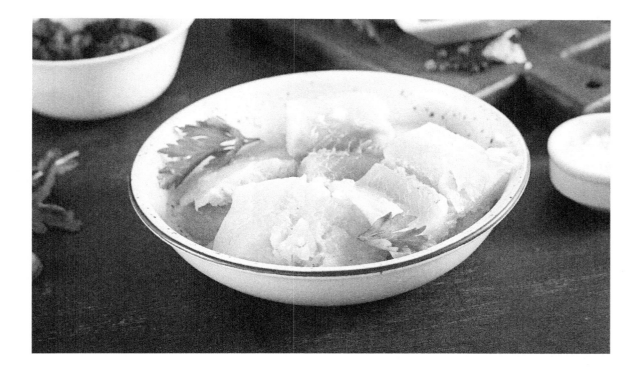

An Italian Christmas tradition is to serve a salad dish made with salted cod. This version replaces the cod with cauliflower while staying true to all the other fabulous flavors.

Servings: 2-4

Total Time: 20mins

Ingredients:

- 1 cauliflower (cut into florets)
- ½ tsp Old Bay seasoning
- 1 (3 ounce) jar capers
- 1 cup Kalamata olives (pitted)
- 1 cup arugula (chopped)
- 1-2 garlic cloves (peeled and minced)
- ½ tsp dulse flakes
- Sea salt (to season)

Dressing:

- ¼ cup extra-virgin olive oil
- Juice of 1 ½ lemons

Directions:

1. Preheat the oven to 400 degrees F.

2. Arrange the cauliflower florets on a baking sheet lined with parchment paper.

3. Scatter the Old Bay seasoning over the cauliflower and roast for approximately 12-15 minutes, until just browned.

4. Take the roasted florets out of the oven and allow to cool.

5. While the roasted cauliflower cools, prepare the dressing.

6. In a bowl, combine the olive oil with the fresh lemon juice, stirring to combine.

7. In a large mixing bowl, combine the cauliflower with the capers, olives, arugula, and dulse flakes.

8. Add the dressing and mix well to combine.

9. Season with sea salt and serve at room temperature.

Creamy No-Clam Chowder

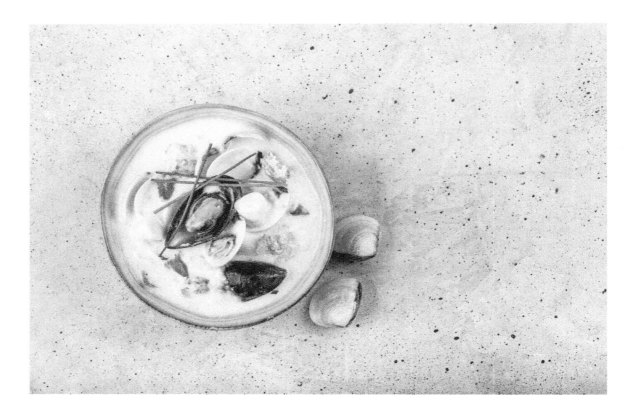

Recreate a creamy clam chowder, but this time, cruelty-free. This plant-based seafood chowder has a buttery texture, and thanks to a small amount of kelp seasoning its sea-like taste.

Servings: 4

Total Time: 8hours 35mins

Ingredients:

Soup base:

- 1 cup raw cashews (soaked overnight)
- 2 medium red potatoes (cut into cubes)
- ½ cup plain soy creamer
- 1 cup plain soy milk
- 1 cup fresh water
- ⅓ cup nutritional yeast
- ½ small yellow onion (peeled and diced)
- ½ tsp kosher salt
- ¼-½ tsp kelp granule seasoning
- ¼ tsp ground black pepper
- ¼ tsp paprika
- ¼ tsp dried oregano
- ¼ tsp powdered garlic
- Freshly squeezed juice of 1 lemon
- Splash of liquid smoke

Mushroom Confit:

- 2 tsp olive oil
- 10 ounces shiitake mushrooms (chopped small)
- ½ cup celery (chopped)
- ½ small yellow onion (peeled and minced)
- 1 garlic clove (peeled and minced)
- Pinch of kosher salt

- Splash of liquid smoke

Directions:

1. Rinse and drain the soaked cashews.

2. Add the potatoes to a microwave-safe bowl and cover with kitchen wrap.

3. Microwave the potatoes on high for approximately 5 minutes, until fork-tender. Set the potatoes to one side until needed.

4. Add the soup base ingredients (cashews, red potatoes, soy creamer, soy milk, water, nutritional yeast, yellow onion, kosher salt, kelp seasoning, black pepper, paprika, dried oregano, powdered garlic, lemon juice, and a splash of liquid smoke. Process on high until the mixture is silky and smooth. Add a drop more water if needed to achieve your desired consistency. Transfer to a pan and on low, heat, while occasionally whisking.

5. Next, prepare the confit. In a sauté pan over moderate heat, heat the oil.

6. Add the chopped mushrooms to the pan, followed by the celery, onion, and garlic and sauté for approximately 5 minutes, increasing the heat to moderate-high.

7. Just before you have finished cooking, season with salt and liquid smoke and stir well to combine. The confit is ready when the celery is softened, and the mushrooms and onions are cooked through.

8. Ladle the chowder into bowls.

9. Spoon the confit into the center of the chowder and serve.

Crockpot Crab-Style Rangoon

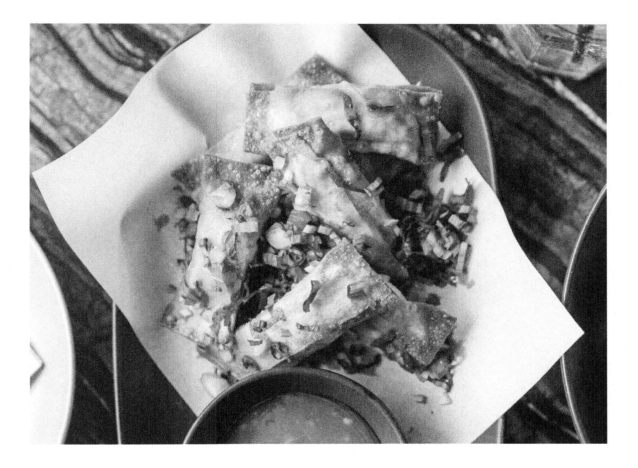

It's not unusual for Chinese take-outs to prepare this dish using a combination of imitation crab meat and cream cheese, which is then deep-fried. Here, by switching some of the ingredients to vegan-friendly options and baking rather than frying, you can create a healthy appetizer or meal.

Servings: 30

Total Time: 2hours 45mins

Ingredients:

- 1 (20 ounce) can young green jackfruit in water (drained)
- 2 cups vegetable broth
- 1 scallion (thinly sliced)
- 2 tsp toasted sesame oil
- 8 ounces cream cheese (room temperature)
- Square wonton wrappers
- Canola oil
- Thai chili sauce (to serve)
- Black and white sesame seeds

Directions:

1. Add the jackfruit and vegetable broth to a crockpot. Push the jackfruit down to make sure it is covered by the broth. If it isn't, you may need to add more. Cook on high, for 2-3 hours.

2. Take the jackfruit out of the broth and shred finely. Remove any tough pieces or seeds. Measure out 1 cup of the shredded jackfruit and place it in a bowl.

3. Add the scallion to the bowl along with the sesame oil and cream cheese - mix well to combine. Put to one side.

4. Preheat the main oven to 425 degrees F.

5. Add 1 teaspoon of the filling into the middle of a wonton. Run a drop of water around the wonton's edges, and fold over to make a triangle. You can do this with your finger.

6. Arrange the wontons on a well-oiled baking tray and bake until golden for 7 minutes. Turn the wantons over and bake on the other side for approximately 4 minutes until golden.

7. Serve with Thai chili sauce and garnish with sesame seeds.

Cruelty-Free Caviar

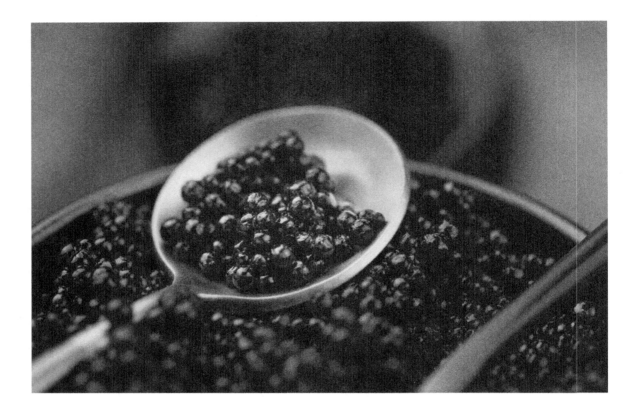

It's good for you, good for the planet, and will help to save the sturgeon from future extinction. What's not to love?

Servings: 8-10

Total Time: 55mins

Ingredients:

- 2 cups extra-virgin olive oil
- 1 cup water
- 2 tbsp ginger (peeled and sliced)
- 2 tbsp dried dulse
- 1 tbsp dried nori
- 1 dehydrated shiitake mushroom
- 1 tbsp caper brine from jar
- 1 tsp soy sauce
- ½ tsp activated charcoal
- 1 tsp agar agar powder

Directions:

1. Pour the oil into a glass bowl and place in the fridge for 45-60 minutes, until cold.

2. Just before you remove the oil from the fridge, bring the water to boil in a small pan. Reduce the heat to low before adding the ginger, dulse, nori, and mushrooms. Rest for 5-10 minutes to steep before removing from the heat. After this time, strain and discard any solids.

3. Return the water to the pan and add the caper brine along with the soy sauce, activated charcoal, and agar-agar. Stir well until the ingredients are dissolved and blended and bring to low heat. Allow to simmer, while stirring for approximately 2-3 minutes while it thickens. Take the pan off the heat.

4. Using a dropper, drip the liquid into the now chilled oil from Step 1. Continue to drip until all the liquid is used. If the mixture in the pan is too solid, add 1 tablespoon or so of cold water and stir to return to liquid form.

5. Strain the oil and store the imitation caviar in the fridge until you ready to enjoy.

Fake Filet-O-Fish

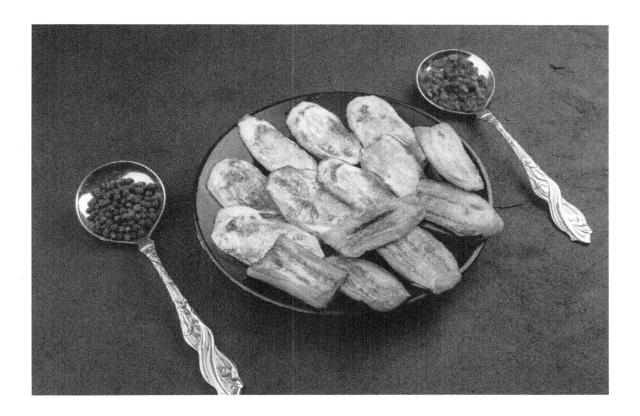

If you prefer, you can switch the eggs for a vegan egg substitute and opt for other vegan-friendly ingredients.

Servings: 1

Total Time: 1hour 15mins

Ingredients:

- 2-3 cups water
- 1 eggplant (peeled and sliced into ½ "square slices)
- ½ cup flour
- 3 eggs
- 1 cup panko breadcrumbs
- 1 hamburger bun
- 1 tbsp prepared tartar sauce
- 1 slice cheese
- Oil (for frying)

Directions:

1. In a casserole dish, combine salt with 2-3 cups of water.

2. Arrange the eggplant slices in the casserole dish and submerge in the water. Soak the eggplant for a minimum of 1 hour.

3. Next, prepare the batter. Using 3 shallow bowls, add flour to the first, the eggs to the second, and breadcrumbs to the third.

4. Preheat your deep-fryer to 375-400 degrees F.

5. Bread the eggplant by dipping each slice first in the flour, then the egg, and finally the breadcrumbs, making sure they are evenly and well coated on both sides. Fry the eggplants on each side for 3-5 minutes, until golden.

6. Steam the bun until it is soft and fluffy.

7. Spread the tartar sauce to the crown side of the hamburger bun.

8. Place the fried eggplant on top, followed by 1 slice of cheese.

9. Add the top of the bun and serve.

Faux-Fish Pie

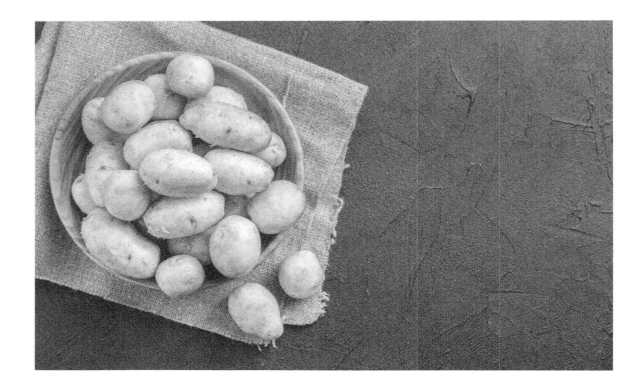

If you are looking for a protein and fiber-rich meal, then add this faux fish pie to your family's weekly menu plan.

Servings: 4

Total Time: 1hour

Ingredients:

Sauce:

- 1 tbsp olive oil
- 1 leek (finely sliced)
- 1 small fennel bulb (tops cut off and coarsely chopped)
- 1 carrot (peeled and coarsely chopped)
- Splash of white wine
- ¾ cup unsweetened cashew milk
- 1 tbsp cornflour
- A handful of fresh dill (coarsely chopped)
- 1 tsp capers (coarsely chopped)
- 1 (14 ounce) can white beans (drained and rinsed)
- A few handfuls of kale
- Salt and black pepper

Potatoes:

- 2 pounds potatoes (peeled and cubed small)
- A handful of fresh dill (coarsely chopped)
- A handful of watercress (coarsely chopped)
- 2 tbsp nutritional yeast
- Salt and black pepper

Directions:

1. In a pan for the sauce, heat the oil until hot.

2. Add the leek along with the fennel and carrots and fry until softened for approximately 10 minutes.

3. Add a splash of white wine and fry for 2-3 minutes until evaporated entirely.

4. Pour the milk into a jug and add the cornflour, stirring to combine.

5. Pour the slurry into the pan and add the dill, capers, beans, and kale. Season the mixture with salt and black pepper and stir well to combine. Bring to boil and while stirring regularly cook until the sauce is thickened.

6. For the potatoes: Add the potatoes to a pan and season with a pinch of salt. Pour in sufficient water to partially cover.

7. Bring the potatoes to boil and on low heat simmer for approximately 15 minutes, until fork-tender. Drain the water and leave the potatoes in the pan.

8. To the potatoes, add the dill, watercress, and yeast. Season the potatoes with salt and black pepper. Using a masher, mash the potatoes until creamy smooth.

9. Preheat the main oven to 350 degrees F.

10. Transfer the sauce to a large casserole dish and spoon over the mash.

11. Using a metal fork, fluff the mash-up to help the potatoes to crisp.

12. Bake the pie in the oven until the top is golden and the sauce bubbles, for 30-40 minutes.

Faux Smoked "Fish" Paté

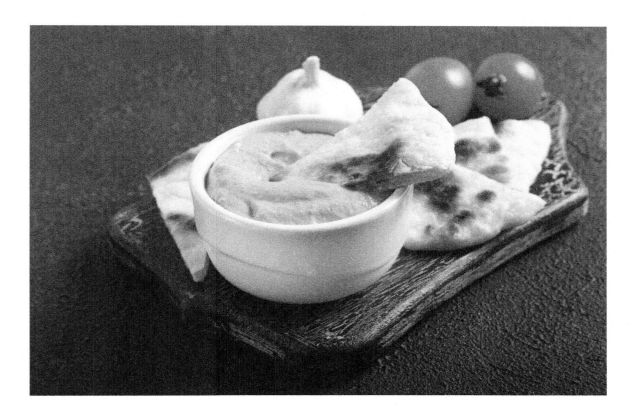

Enjoy this faux-fish paté with chunks of crusty baguette. It's easy to prepare, healthy, and no fish were harmed during its preparation!

Servings: 2

Total Time: 12mins

Ingredients:

- 1½ cups canned beans, of choice (drained and rinsed)
- 1 tsp smoked oil
- 2-3 drop liquid smoke
- 1 tsp dairy-free plain yogurt
- 1 tsp capers in brine (coarsely chopped)
- 1 tsp freshly squeezed lemon juice
- 1 tsp dulse powder
- Salt and black pepper
- Parsley (chopped, to garnish)
- Crusty bread (to serve, optional)

Directions:

1. Add the beans, smoked oil, liquid smoke, yogurt, capers, lemon juice, and dulse powder to a bowl and with a fork, mash, leaving some texture.

2. Season the paté with salt and black pepper and garnish with chopped parsley.

3. Serve with crusty bread.

Fish-Free Sushi

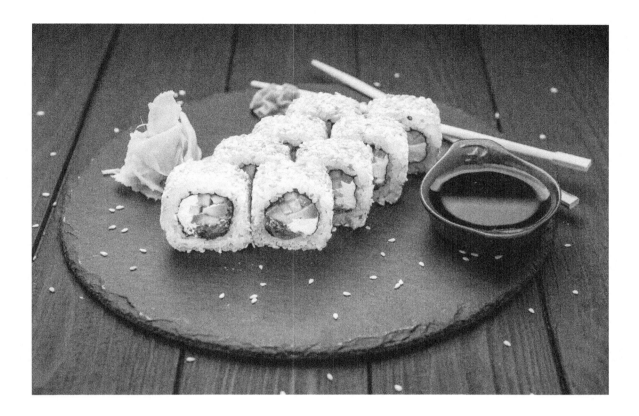

Just because you're skipping seafood doesn't mean you have to miss out on this Japanese delicacy. Make your own sushi using fresh vegetables for a fun and interactive meal to share with friends.

Servings: 24

Total Time: 15mins

Ingredients:

Sushi:

- 2 nori sheets (cut in half)
- 8 ounces cooked brown sushi rice
- ½ cucumber (deseeded, julienned)
- ½ red bell pepper (deseeded, julienned)
- ½ avocado (peeled, destoned, julienned)

Dipping Sauce:

- 3 tbsp soy sauce
- Juice of 1 lime
- 3 tbsp mirin
- Small bunch spring onions (diced)
- 2 tbsp wasabi
- 2 tbsp pickled ginger

Directions:

1. Arrange the nori sheets on a sushi mat, shiny side down. Spoon half the cooked rice on top of the nori and spread into an even layer leaving a 1" strip of nori free at the top.

2. Make a hollow well in the center of the rice and arrange the julienned cucumber, bell pepper, or avocado in the well.

3. Starting from the end closest to you, roll the nori carefully so as not to push out the filling. Cut the nori roll into 1" slices using a serrated knife.

4. Repeat with the remaining ingredients.

5. Transfer the sushi to a serving platter and arrange in an attractive design.

6. Prepare the sauce. Add the soy sauce, lime juice, mirin, and spring onions to a small bowl and arrange on the platter for dipping.

7. Arrange the wasabi and pickled ginger on the platter in a small mound and serve.

Gefilte "Fish"

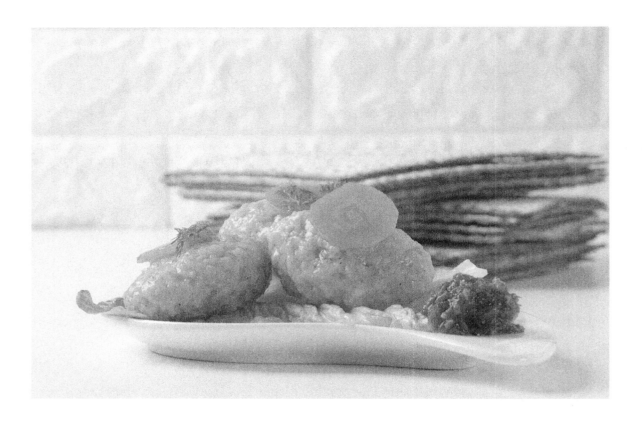

This classic Kosher Passover dish gets a plant-based seafood makeover with tasty vegetables and fresh ingredients.

Servings: 4

Total Time: 1hour 30mins

Ingredients:

- 3 potatoes (peeled)
- Canola oil
- 2 yellow onions (peeled and diced)
- 1 eggplant (topped and tailed, halved lengthwise)
- 2 tbsp fresh parsley (chopped)
- 2 garlic cloves (peeled and minced)
- Sea salt and black pepper
- Smoked paprika
- Matzah meal (as needed)

Directions:

1. Boil the potatoes in salted water until tender. Drain and set to one side.

2. Preheat the main oven to 425 degrees F.

3. Warm a drop of oil in a skillet over moderately high heat. Add the onion and sauté for 3-4 minutes until softened. Take off the heat.

4. Brush the eggplant halves with a little oil and arrange on a baking sheet cut side down. Prick the eggplant skin a few times and then place it in the oven. Cook for approximately 25 minutes until the flesh is soft. Scoop the flesh from the skin and transfer to a bowl.

5. Turn the oven temperature down to 350 degrees F and grease a baking sheet with oil.

6. Mash the cooked potatoes and transfer to a bowl along with the sautéed onion, eggplant flesh, parsley, and garlic—season to taste with salt, black pepper, and smoked paprika.

7. Mix in just enough matzah meal to give a firm, shapeable consistency.

8. Taking tablespoonfuls of the mixture, shape into patties and place on the greased baking sheet. Sprinkle the top of the patties with a drop of oil.

9. Place in the oven and bake for half an hour until golden. Serve warm.

Hearts of Palm Calamari

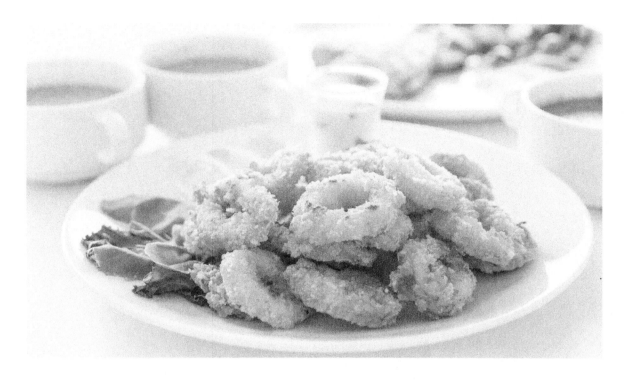

Serve this fish-free fried calamari at your next party or get-together. Your guests will be amazed at just how like the real thing this appetizer tastes.

Servings: 3-4

Total Time: 30mins

Ingredients:

Cocktail Sauce:

- ¼ cup ketchup
- 2 tsp horseradish, store-bought
- Freshly squeezed juice of ½ lemon
- ½ tsp pepper
- Salt (to season)

Batter:

- 1½ cups tempura mix
- 1-2 cups chilled water
- 3 nori seaweed sheets (finely ground)
- ½ tsp sea salt
- ½ tsp freshly ground black pepper

Calamari:

- 2 (14 ounce) cans hearts of palm (drained)
- 1½ cups all-purpose flour
- 1 tbsp Old Bay seasoning
- 1 tbsp fish seasoning
- Lemon wedges (to serve)

Directions:

1. For the cocktail sauce: In a bowl, combine the ketchup with the horseradish, lemon juice, and pepper. Taste and season with salt before transferring to the fridge to chill until needed.

2. For the batter: Add the tempura mix to a mixing bowl.

3. Stir in the water slowly to create a pancake batter-like consistency.

4. Stir in the ground seaweed and season with salt and pepper. Put the bowl to one side.

5. For the calamari: First, cut each heart of palm into equal halves. Using a straw, gently push out the soft center to leave a hollow barrel.

6. Slice each barrel into rings, approximately 1" thick, to resemble calamari rings.

7. In a ziplock bag, combine the flour with the Old Bay seasoning and fish seasoning. Seal and shake the bag to combine.

8. In batches, add the calamari first in the batter and then in the flour mixture in the plastic bag. Gently toss the bag to evenly and thoroughly coat.

9. Over moderate to high heat, in a frying pan, add the rings to the oil. Fry until crisp and golden, for 2-3 minutes.

10. Using a slotted spoon, remove the rings from the oil and transfer to a plate lined with kitchen paper towels.

11. Serve alongside the cocktail sauce with fresh lemon wedges.

Jackfruit 'Crab' Cakes

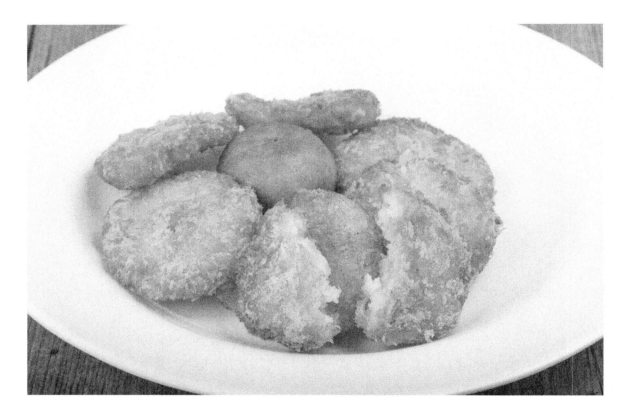

Cruelty-free cakes are all about the taste and texture. Enjoy as an appetizer, side, or main with your favorite dip.

Servings: 6

Total Time: 25mins

Ingredients

- 2 tbsp ground flax seed
- 6 tbsp water
- 1 tsp yellow mustard
- 1 tbsp freshly squeezed lemon juice
- 1 tsp Worcestershire sauce
- 24 ounces young jackfruit in water (drained, rinsed, squeezed, patted dry, chopped)
- 2 tbsp Old Bay seasoning
- 2 cloves of garlic (peeled and minced)
- 1 tsp ground sea salt
- ½ tsp freshly ground black pepper
- 3 tbsp chives (minced)
- ¼ cup cilantro (minced)
- ½ cup regular breadcrumbs
- ½ cup panko breadcrumbs
- Lemon wedges

Directions:

1. First, make the flax eggs by combining the ground flaxseed with the water and setting aside to sit for 10 minutes.

2. Add the mustard, fresh lemon juice, and Worcestershire sauce to a large bowl, and whisk to incorporate fully.

3. Add the jackfruit, flax egg, Old Bay seasoning, garlic, sea salt, black pepper, chives, cilantro, breadcrumbs, and panko breadcrumbs to a bowl and using clean hands, combine. Once the mixture adheres to itself, form it into 6 patties.

4. Place the patties on a plate and transfer to the fridge for a minimum of 30 minutes.

5. Preheat the main oven to 375 degrees F.

6. Remove the patties from the fridge and arrange on a baking sheet.

7. Squeeze fresh lemon juice over the top of the cakes and bake for 10-12 minutes, until golden. Flip over, squeeze with lemon juice and bake until golden brown and firm.

8. Serve and enjoy.

King Oyster Scallop Cioppino

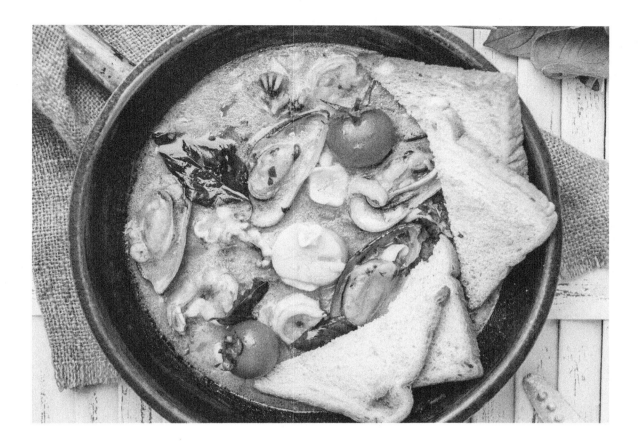

This classic Italian stew is seasoned to perfection. Better yet, King Oyster mushrooms replace its usual seafood without sacrificing texture or taste.

Servings: 2-4

Total Time: 45mins

Ingredients:

- 8 ounces King Oyster mushrooms (stalks cut into 1½" thick rounds)
- 1 tbsp butter
- 1 tbsp olive oil
- ¼ cup celery (thinly sliced)
- ¼ cup yellow onion (peeled and diced small)
- 4 garlic cloves (peeled and thinly sliced)
- 1 (14½ ounce) can garbanzo beans (rinsed and drained)
- 4 Roma tomatoes (diced)
- 1½ cups vegetable broth
- 1 tsp Old Bay seasoning
- ¼ freshly squeezed lemon juice
- 2 tbsp fresh parsley (chopped and divided)
- Salt (to season)
- Freshly ground black pepper (to season)

Directions:

1. Add the mushrooms to a bowl, and fill with sufficient hot water, to cover. Soak the mushrooms for 5 minutes before draining and patting dry.

2. Over moderate-high heat, melt the butter in a large frying pan.

3. Once melted, add the mushrooms, and cook for 3-4 minutes until gently browned.

4. Flip the mushrooms over and cook on the other side for an additional 3-4 minutes until gently browned. Take the pan off the heat and cover with a lid to keep warm.

5. Over moderate to high heat, in a large pot heat the olive oil.

6. Add the celery along with the onion and cook for 3-5 minutes, while frequently sitting until just softened. Add the garlic and cook for 60 seconds.

7. Add the beans followed by the tomatoes, broth, and Old Bay seasoning.

8. Turn the heat down to low and simmer for approximately 15 minutes.

9. Stir in the fresh lemon juice and 1 tablespoon of parsley. Taste the cioppino and season with salt and black pepper.

10. Ladle the cioppino into bowls and top with the mushroom 'scallops'.

11. Garnish with the remaining parsley and serve.

Lobster Mushroom Bisque

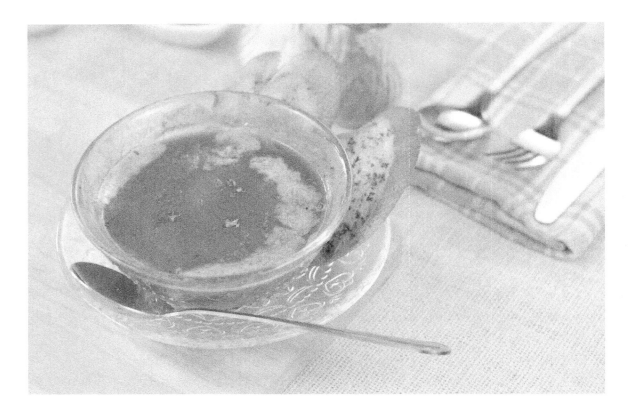

Lobster mushrooms are a reddish-orange color, and they look a lot like the outer shell of a cooked lobster, which makes them an ideal ingredient for this delicious seafood-free bisque.

Servings: 6

Total Time: 40mins

Ingredients:

- 1 cup raw cashews (soaked in water overnight)
- 6 cups vegetable broth (divided)
- 1 tbsp kelp powder
- 1 tbsp cornstarch
- 2 cups dried Lobster mushrooms (soaked and diced)
- 2 tbsp olive oil
- 2 cups onion (peeled and minced)
- 4 cloves of garlic (peeled and crushed)
- 4 large celery ribs (diced small)
- 2 carrots (diced small)
- 2 tbsp tomato paste
- 1 cup dry white wine
- 1 tsp smoked paprika
- 1 tsp thyme
- Pinch of cayenne
- 1 bay leaf
- Salt and freshly ground black pepper (to season)
- Parsley leaves (minced, to garnish)

Directions:

1. Drain the soaked cashews.

2. Add the soaked cashews to a food blender along with 1 cup of vegetable broth, kelp powder, and cornstarch. Process until smooth, this step will take 2-3 minutes. Put to one side.

3. According to the package instructions, soak the lobster mushrooms, setting ¼ cup aside for garnishing. Soaking is usually around 10 minutes.

4. Add the oil to a stockpot and set over moderate heat.

5. Add the onion followed by the garlic, celery, and carrots to the pot and cook until softened, for 3-4 minutes.

6. Stir in the tomato paste and cook for a couple of minutes before adding the wine to deglaze the pan. Simmer for approximately 2 minutes.

7. Add the broth, cashew mixture, smoked paprika, thyme, cayenne, and bay leaf. Season with salt and black pepper. Bring the mixture to simmer, turn the heat down to low and cook for approximately 10 minutes.

8. Remove and discard the bay leaf from the bisque.

9. In batches, puree the mixture until silky smooth.

10. Return the bisque to the pot and add the diced mushrooms. Simmer for 3-5 minutes, until heated through.

11. Ladle into serving bowls and garnish each portion with parsley.

Lobster Mushroom Fra Diavolo

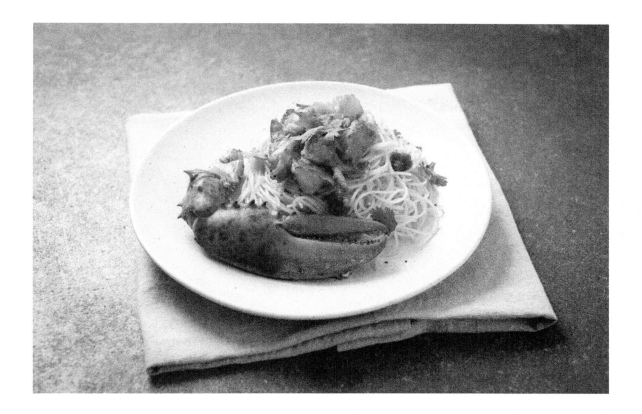

Lobster mushrooms not only look a little like lobster but taste like it too, which is great news for lobster lovers who are looking to reduce their impact on nature and the environment.

Servings: 4

Total Time: 10mins

Ingredients:

- 2 ounces dried lobster mushrooms (rehydrated as per packet instructions)
- 1 tbsp olive oil
- 5 garlic cloves (peeled and sliced thinly)
- 12 ounces marinara sauce
- ¾ tsp crushed red pepper flakes
- 1½ cups vegetable stock
- ½ cup dry white wine
- 8 ounces spaghetti

Directions:

1. Rinse the rehydrated lobster mushrooms and set them to one side.

2. Warm the olive oil in a pan over moderate heat. Add the garlic and sauté for 3-4 minutes until golden.

3. Pour in the marinara sauce and season with crushed red pepper flakes. Bring to a simmer for a few minutes and then take off the heat.

4. In a second pan, bring the vegetable stock and dry white wine to a simmer over moderately low heat. Add the set-aside mushrooms and cook for half an hour.

5. Cook the spaghetti using packet instructions, drain and return to the pot.

6. Pour the mushrooms and stock into the marinara sauce and stir well. Pour the mixture over the pasta and toss to combine.

7. Divide between bowls and serve straight away.

Lobster Mushroom Mac 'n Cheese

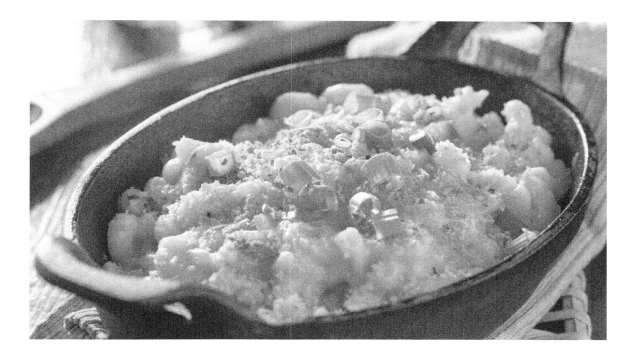

Give this classic Mac 'n Cheese recipe a seafood-free makeover with vibrant lobster mushrooms and cashew-based sauce.

Servings: 6

Total Time: 1hour 40mins

Ingredients:

- 1 ounce dried lobster mushrooms (soaked overnight, soaking liquid reserved)

Sauce:

- 1 cup raw cashews
- ¾ cup water
- 2 tbsp coconut oil (melted)
- 2 tbsp plum vinegar
- 2 tbsp nutritional yeast
- 1 tbsp roasted garlic (mashed)
- 1 tbsp freshly squeezed lemon juice
- 1 tbsp mellow white miso
- ⅛ tsp salt

Pasta:

- ½ pound uncooked spiral pasta
- 1½ tbsp olive oil (divided)
- 3 shallots (thinly sliced)
- Salt
- ¼ cup mushroom soaking liquid (strained well)
- ¾ cup water
- 2 tbsp breadcrumbs

Directions:

1. Preheat the main oven to 350 degrees F. Put a casserole or baking dish on a half sheet pan.

2. For the mushrooms: Remove them from the water and set the liquid aside. Squeeze to drain and add to a mesh strainer. Rinse under cold running water to remove any debris or grit. Chop the mushrooms into bite-size pieces and put to one side.

3. Strain the set aside soaking water through a kitchen paper towel and put it to one side.

4. Make the sauce. In a food blender, blend the cashews with the water until silky smooth. Next, add the oil, nutritional yeast, vinegar, roasted garlic, fresh lemon juice, miso, and salt to the blender. Process until smooth and put aside.

5. For the pasta: Bring a large pan of salted water to boil. Cook the pasta according to the package directions. Set some cooking water aside. Drain the pasta and return it to the pan.

6. Over moderately low heat, in a skillet, warm 1 tablespoon of oil. Once the oil shimmers, add the shallots and season with salt, cooking for 5 minutes, until translucent.

7. Next, add the mushrooms and stir.

8. Pour in the mushroom soaking liquid and water and bring to simmer. Uncovered, cook while occasionally stirring until the majority of the liquid has evaporated and the mushrooms are softened, for approximately half an hour.

9. Pour the mushroom and shallot mixture along with the prepared sauce into the pasta pot. Gently stir to combine, adding a drop of pasta water, if need to make a silky sauce. Pour the mixture into the preheated baking dish.

10. In a bowl, combine the breadcrumbs with the remaining oil, stirring until combined entirely. Scatter the crumb mixture on top of the Mac 'n Cheese and bake in the preheated oven for half an hour. The dish is ready when the top is crisp, and the sauce is gently bubbling.

11. Allow to stand for 10-15 minutes and serve.

Mexican-Style 'Seafood' Stew

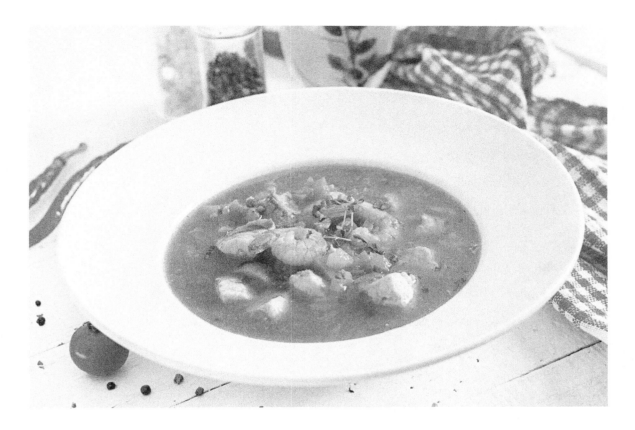

This Mexican-style stew is spicy and tangy. It features oyster mushrooms, garbanzo beans, hearts of palm, and corn simmered in a chili-tomato broth. Enjoy all your favorite garnishes, including cilantro, fresh lime, and tostadas.

Servings: 8

Total Time: 1hour

Ingredients:

- 2 tbsp vegetable oil (divided)
- 4 garlic cloves (peeled and minced)
- ½ tbsp dried Mexican oregano
- 1 tsp sea salt
- ½ tsp black pepper
- 2 tsp ground cumin
- 2 tsp ancho chili powder
- 1 tsp chipotle powder
- 2 tbsp nori seaweed (ground)
- 8 dried guajillo chilies (soaked, seeded, and chopped)
- 4 Roma tomatoes (roasted and peeled)
- 8 ounces tomato sauce
- 2 carrots (cut into medium dice)
- 1 medium onion (peeled and diced)
- 3 stalks celery (chopped into medium dice)
- 8 ounces oyster mushrooms (separated)
- 4 cups vegetable stock
- 14 ounces hearts of palm (half diced into rings, half julienned)
- 4 ears fresh corn on the cob (snapped into halves)
- 1½ cups garbanzo beans (rinsed, drained and cooked)
- ½ cup cilantro, chopped (to garnish)
- Fresh lime wedges (to garnish)
- Tostados (to serve, optional)

Directions:

1. In a large soup pot, heat 1 tablespoon of oil.

2. To the pot, add the garlic, Mexican oregano, sea salt, black pepper, cumin, chili powder, chipotle powder, ground nori, and sauté for 3 minutes.

3. Next, add the rehydrated chilies, tomatoes, and tomato sauce. Reduce the heat and simmer for 10 minutes.

4. For the soup base, puree the mixture and transfer to a bowl. Put to one side.

5. Using the same pot, heat the remaining oil on moderate heat and sauté the veggies (carrots, onions, celery, and mushrooms) for 3-5 minutes.

6. Return the soup base to the pot and pour in the vegetable stock. Cook the mixture for approximately 10 minutes.

7. Next, add the hearts of palm along with the corn and garbanzo beans, cook for 5-6 minutes.

8. Serve the stew hot garnished with chopped cilantro and wedges of fresh lime.

9. Enjoy with tostadas.

Mushroom Stuffed Clams

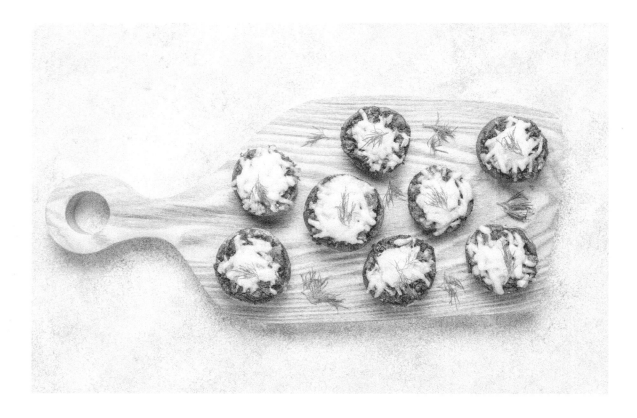

This delicious dish of mushrooms stuffed clams presented on a serving board is the perfect show-stopping appetizer to serve family and friends.

Servings: 4

Total Time: 45mins

Ingredients:

- 8 ounces shiitake mushrooms (sliced)
- 1 tbsp soy sauce
- 1 cup Italian-style breadcrumbs
- Juice of 2 lemons
- 1 cup vegetable broth
- Handful fresh parsley (chopped)
- ¼ cup Parmesan cheese (grated)
- 1 tbsp olive oil
- 1 garlic clove (peeled and minced)
- ½ tsp dulse flakes
- ¼ tsp Old Bay seasoning
- Paprika
- Empty clamshells
- Lemon wedges

Directions:

1. Preheat the main oven to 400 degrees F. Cover a baking sheet with parchment paper.

2. Add the mushrooms to a bowl and drizzle over the soy sauce, toss to coat, then transfer to the baking sheet in an even layer.

3. Place in the oven and bake for 15-20 minutes. Take out of the oven and allow to cool before chopping into smaller pieces. Set to one side.

4. Turn the oven temperature down to 350 degrees F.

5. Combine the breadcrumbs, lemon juice, vegetable broth, parsley, Parmesan cheese, olive oil, garlic, dulse flakes, Old Bay seasoning, and pinch of paprika.

6. Add the mushrooms to the breadcrumbs mixture and toss to combine.

7. Stuff the mushroom mixture into empty clam shells and arrange the stuffed shells on a baking sheet.

8. Place in the oven and bake for 15 minutes until golden.

9. Transfer to a serving board and garnish with lemon wedges.

'No-Tuna' Salad Whole-Wheat Sandwiches

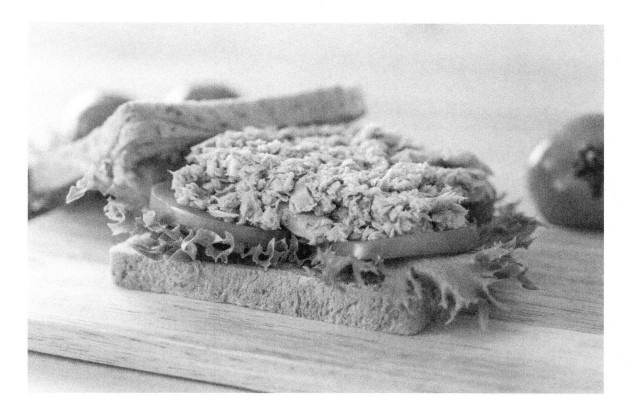

These vegan tuna sandwiches are delicious. They are easy to make and taste a lot like the seafood version.

Servings: 4

Total Time: 10mins

Ingredients:

- 1 (15-ounce) can garbanzo beans (rinsed and drained)
- 3 tbsp tahini
- 1 tsp Dijon mustard
- 1 tbsp maple syrup
- ¼ cup red onion (peeled and diced)
- ¼ cup celery (trimmed and diced)
- ¼ cup dill pickle (diced)
- Sea salt and freshly ground black pepper
- 1 tbsp roasted sunflower seeds
- 8 slices whole-wheat bread
- Romaine lettuce (torn, to serve)
- Tomato, sliced (to serve)
- Red onion (peeled and sliced, to serve)

Directions:

1. Add the garbanzo beans to a mixing bowl and with a fork, mash leaving only a few beans whole.

2. Add the tahini to the bowl along with the Dijon mustard, maple syrup, onion, celery, and pickle. Season with salt and black pepper. Next, add the sunflower seeds, and mix to combine.

3. Toast the bread.

4. Add the lettuce, tomato slices, and red onion.

5. Divide the filling between 4 slices of the toasted bread and spoon on top.

6. Top with the toasted bread to create 4 sandwiches.

Oven-Fried Faux-Fish Sticks

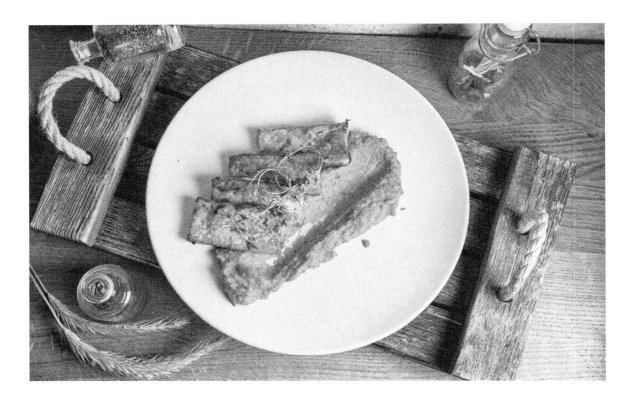

Oven-fried faux fish sticks are crunchy and crisp. Better yet, your children will love them too! They make the perfect after-school meal.

Servings: 4

Total Time: 1hour 30mins

Ingredients:

Marinade:

- 2 tbsp low-sodium soy sauce
- Juice of ½ lime
- ½ cup dulse powder
- 1 tsp Old Bay seasoning
- ½ cup water

Tofu:

- 14 ounces extra-firm tofu (drained and pressed for 30mins)
- ½ cup unsweetened almond milk
- 2 eggs
- 1 tbsp fresh lemon juice
- ¼ cup flour
- ½ cup breadcrumbs
- ¼ tsp cayenne pepper
- ½ tsp salt
- ¼ tsp black pepper
- ½ tsp garlic powder
- ½ tsp onion powder
- 1 tbsp nutritional yeast
- Tartar sauce (to serve)
- Vinegar (to serve)
- Lemon wedges (to serve)
- Parsley (minced)

Directions:

1. Preheat the main oven to 400 degrees F.

2. For the marinade: In a bowl, combine the soy sauce with the fresh lime juice, dulse, Old Bay seasoning, and water. Stir well to combine, and transfer to the fridge for 20 minutes.

3. After this, add the tofu to the marinade and marinate for 60 minutes.

4. In a shallow dish, combine the almond milk, eggs, and lemon juice.

5. In a second shallow dish, combine the flour with the breadcrumbs, cayenne pepper, salt, black pepper, garlic powder, onion powder, and nutritional yeast.

6. Remove the tofu from the marinade and slice lengthwise into ½" sticks.

7. Dunk the stick first in the wet mixture and then dredge in the breadcrumb mixture.

8. Place the sticks on a lightly oiled sheet of parchment paper, set on a baking sheet.

9. Bake in the preheated oven for approximately 15 minutes, on each side, until crunchy and brown.

10. Serve with optional tartar sauce, vinegar, lemon wedges, and parsley.

Oyster Mushroom 'Scallop' Pasta with White Wine Sauce

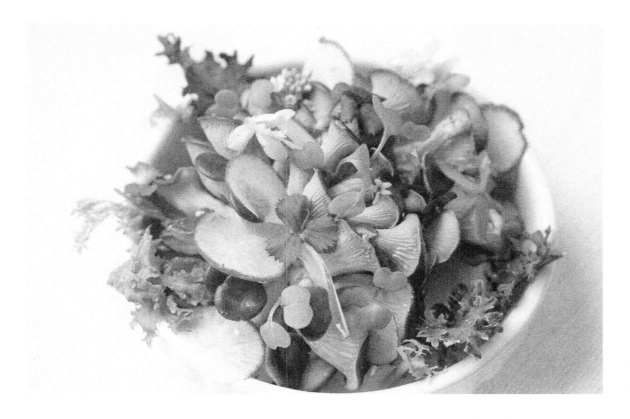

You can recreate the texture of fresh scallops quite easily by switching them for pre-soaked mushroom stems. Enjoy!

Servings: 2

Total Time: 1hour

Ingredients:

- Splash of olive oil (for pasta water)
- Sea salt (as needed)
- 2 cups bow tie pasta
- 2 tbsp nut butter
- 1 shallot (sliced thinly)
- 4 garlic cloves (peeled and minced)
- ⅓ cup white wine
- ⅔ cup vegetable broth
- 1 tbsp canned coconut milk cream*
- ⅓ cup fresh parsley (chopped, divided)
- 1 tbsp fresh lemon zest (divided)
- 4 king oyster mushroom stems (sliced, soaked in warm water for 30-60 minutes)
- 1-2 tbsp capers
- Freshly cracked pepper

Directions:

1. Bring a pot of water to boil. Add a splash of oil and a few pinches of salt to the water and cook the bow-tie pasta until al dente.

2. In the meantime, prepare the sauce.

3. In a skillet, melt 1 tablespoon of nut butter over moderate heat. Add the shallot and a few more pinches of salt. Stir well to coat and sauté for approximately 3 minutes.

4. Next, add the garlic and sauté for an additional 2 minutes.

5. Turn the heat up to high and after 60 seconds; pour in the wine and allow it to sizzle for 30 seconds or so. Reduce the heat to moderate and pour in the broth.

6. Next, stir in the coconut cream followed by half of the parsley and half of the lemon zest.

7. Once the pasta is al dente, drain and add it to the sauce, stir well to incorporated and allow to simmer on the lowest possible heat while you prepare the faux scallops.

8. In a clean frying pan, melt the remaining nut butter over moderate heat.

9. Remove the mushrooms out from the water, and without drying them, add them to the frying pan. Cover the pan and allow them to soften for several minutes.

10. Take the lid of the pan and allow the liquid to evaporate entirely and the mushroom to develop a light caramelized color on all sides. Remove the mushrooms from the heat and spoon them into the pasta and sauce. Toss the mixture well to coat evenly.

11. Transfer to a serving bowl and garnish with the remaining parsley, lemon zest, and the capers.

12. Season with black pepper and enjoy.

*Skim the cream off the top of a can of coconut milk

Pan-Seared Watermelon Steak

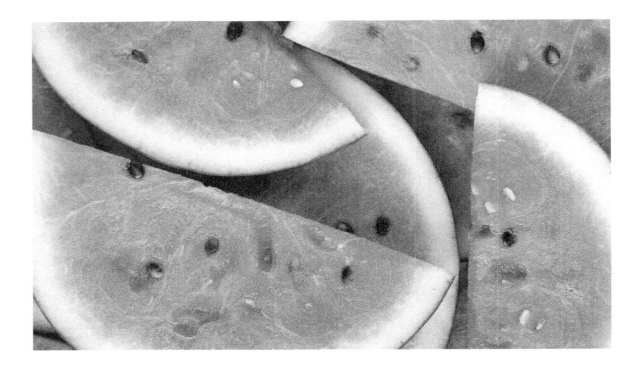

Transform juicy watermelon into tuna-like rare steaks by searing them in a pan. Serve with salty feta cheese and a balsamic reduction.

Servings: 6

Total Time: 30mins

Ingredients:

- ½ cup balsamic vinegar
- ½ large watermelon
- 2 tbsp extra-virgin olive oil
- ½ tsp liquid smoke
- 2 cloves of garlic (peeled and minced)
- ¼ tsp salt
- ¼ tsp freshly ground black pepper
- Feta cheese (crumbled, to serve)
- Fresh mint (chopped, to serve)

Directions:

1. In a small pan, bring ½ cup of balsamic vinegar to simmer. Whisk the vinegar occasionally, allowing it to cook and reduce to a thick and syrup-like consistency that can coat the pan. Set aside until ready to use.

2. Cut the watermelon in half, lengthwise. Place the watermelon flat side facing downwards on a chopping board and cut into 1½" slices. Cut the largest size rectangle you can from each slice. Aim to yield 6 steaks for the watermelon half.

3. Using kitchen paper towels, pat the watermelon steaks dry and transfer to the fridge, uncovered for 1-2 hours. They will need one final pat dry before preparing.

4. In a bowl, whisk the oil with the liquid smoke, garlic, salt, and black pepper. Brush the mixture liberally over both sides of the melon.

5. Over low to moderate heat, lightly grease a sauté pan.

6. Slide each watermelon steak into the pan and cook for approximately 5 minutes on each side.

7. Turn the heat up to moderate to high heat and continue to cook on each side for 60 seconds, until gently brown3ed.

8. Serve warm and top with the balsamic reduction, crumbled feta, and fresh mint.

Plant-Based Shrimp Scampi Linguini

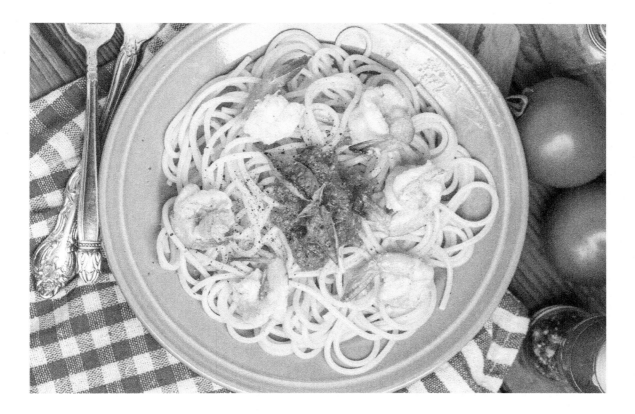

This delicious pasta dish brings together linguine, zucchini, and plant-based scampi cooked in butter and white wine. It's a simple yet classy meal that's perfect for serving the next time you have fellow environment-conscious friends over.

Servings: 4

Total Time: 30mins

Ingredients:

- 9 ounces linguine
- 1 zucchini (spiralized)
- 2 tbsp butter
- 1 onion (peeled, diced)
- 3 garlic cloves (peeled and minced)
- 8½ ounces breaded plant-based shrimp
- Juice of 1 lemon
- ¼ cup dry white wine
- ⅓ cup fresh parsley (chopped)
- Salt and black pepper

Directions:

1. Cook the linguine using packet instructions. For the final 1-2 minutes of cooking, add the zucchini to boiling pasta water. Drain and set to one side.

2. Melt 1 tbsp butter in a skillet over moderate heat. Add the onion and sauté for 2-3 minutes. Next, add the garlic and sauté another 60 seconds. Transfer the onion and garlic to a side plate.

3. Melt the remaining butter in the skillet, add the breaded shrimp and sauté until golden and hot through.

4. Return the onion and garlic to the skillet along with the lemon juice, white wine, and parsley. Increase the heat to moderately high and cook for 60 more seconds until piping hot.

5. Add the linguine and zucchini to the skillet and toss to combine all of the ingredients.

6. Season to taste with salt and black pepper and serve.

'Seafood' Linguine

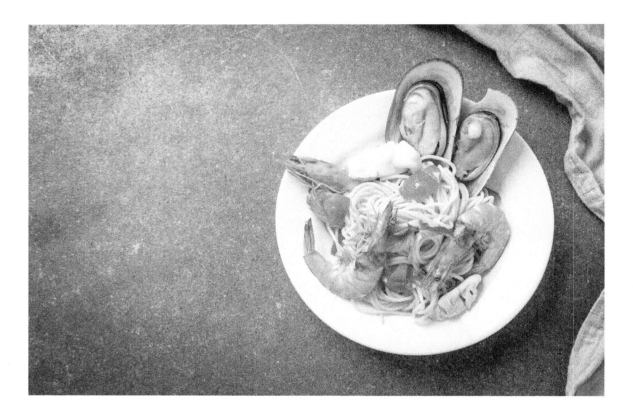

Who doesn't like a delicious linguine? However, what we don't all love is a meal at the expense of ocean life. So, why not opt for this cruelty-free pasta dish made with King Oyster mushrooms.

Servings: 6

Total Time: 30mins

Ingredients:

- Oil (as needed)
- 1 large King Oyster mushrooms (cut into discs)
- Salt and black pepper (to season)
- 12 ounces linguine
- 3 tbsp butter
- 3 garlic cloves (peeled and minced)
- 1 (14 ounce) can hearts of palm (drained and cut into half circles)
- 1 (14 ounce) can banana blossoms (drained and sliced)
- ½ tsp red pepper flakes
- Freshly squeezed juice of 2 lemons
- ½ tsp dried kelp
- A large bunch of fresh parsley leaves (stemmed and leaves coarsely chopped)

Directions:

1. Over moderate to high heat, in a skillet heat a drop of oil.

2. Add the mushrooms to the pan and sear on both sides before seasoning with salt and pepper. Remove the mushrooms from the pan and put to one side.

3. Cook the pasta until al dente. Drain, keep warm, and set aside.

4. In the same pan you used to cook the mushrooms, melt the butter over moderate heat. Add the minced garlic to the pan.

5. Next, add the hearts of palm along with the banana blossoms, red pepper flakes, fresh lemon juice, and kelp. Sauté for 4-5 minutes, while occasionally stirring to combine.

6. Add the seared mushrooms and drained pasta, toss to evenly combine and garnish with chopped parsley.

7. Serve and enjoy.

Spanish-Style Lobster Mushroom Paella

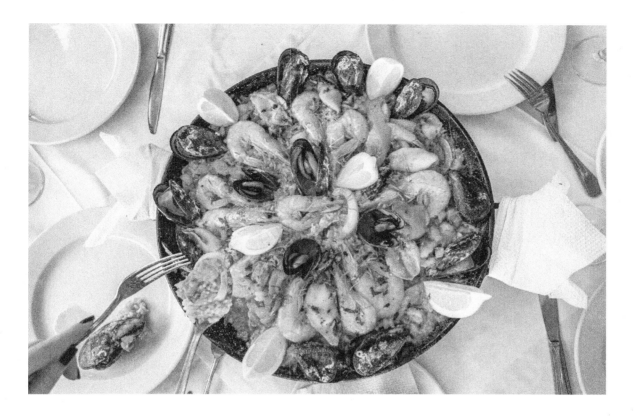

This cruelty-free paella with lobster mushrooms rather than actual lobster not only helps to save the planet but also saves money!

Servings: 4

Total Time: 1hour 15mins

Ingredients:

- 1 tbsp olive oil
- 2 cloves of garlic (peeled and thinly sliced)
- 1 cup jasmine rice
- ½ tsp saffron threads
- ½ cup white wine
- 3 ounces dried lobster mushrooms (soaked in hot water for 30 minutes, drained)
- 2 cups vegetable broth
- 1 tsp smoked paprika
- 2 ounces sundried tomatoes (halved)
- ¾ cup frozen peas

Directions:

1. Over moderate to high heat in a large frying pan, warm the oil.

2. Add the garlic to the pan and sauté until slightly browned and softened.

3. Add the rice to the pan, crumble in the saffron and cook while stirring for 2-3 minutes until the rice grains are well coated.

4. Pour in the wine and cook for 5 minutes, or until the liquid is mostly absorbed.

5. Stir in the mushrooms.

6. Pour in the vegetable broth and stir in the smoked paprika. Bring to boil and reduce the heat to low, cover with a lid and without stirring, cook for 20 minutes, until the rice is mostly absorbed.

7. Add the tomatoes to the pan of rice at the end of its 20 minutes cooking time.

8. In a microwave, heat the peas for a couple of minutes.

9. Transfer the dish to a serving dish or serve straight from the pan.

10. Sprinkle the peas over the top of the paella and add 2-3 lemon slices.

11. Serve and enjoy.

Spicy Seaweed Tofu Rolls

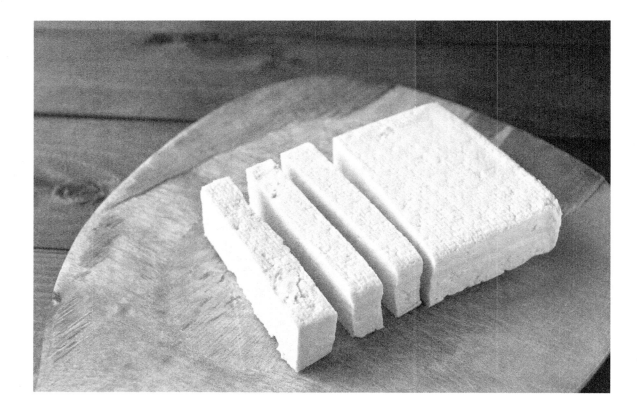

Seaweed-wrapped tofu and sautéed with lemongrass, garlic, and chili, not only healthy, but they are spicy with a great fish-like flavor.

Servings: 6

Total Time: 50mins

Ingredients:

- 8¾ ounces tofu
- 2 tbsp oil
- 2 nori sheets
- 2 tsp flour (diluted in 1 tbsp water)
- 1 garlic clove (peeled and minced)
- ½ lemongrass (minced)
- ½ small chili (finely sliced)
- 1 tbsp soy sauce
- 1 tbsp coconut sugar
- 1 tbsp water
- Freshly squeezed lime juice (to serve)
- Green onions (chopped, to serve)

Directions:

1. Slice the tofu into ½" thick and 2½" long rectangles.

2. Over moderate heat, heat 1 tablespoon of oil in a skillet.

3. When the oil is hot, add the tofu and fry for approximately 5 minutes, or until golden on all sides. Take the pan off the heat and transfer the tofu to a kitchen paper towel-lined plate.

4. Cut the nori sheets into 3 even strips. Slice each strip in half. The sheets should be approximately the same width as the tofu, and sufficiently long enough to wrap.

5. In a small bowl, combine the rice flour in the water and put it aside.

6. Wrap a rectangle of tofu tightly in a nori sheet. Dampen the top slightly of the nori sheet with the rice and flour mixture and continue wrapping. The rice and flour mixture will help to seal the rolls. Repeat the process with the remaining tofu.

7. Over moderate heat, heat a 1 tablespoon of oil in a skillet or frying pan. When hot, add the garlic followed by the lemongrass and chili and sauté for a couple of minutes.

8. Add the tofu rolls to the pan and sauté for an additional 2 minutes, while regularly stirring.

9. In a bowl, combine the soy sauce with the coconut sugar and water.

10. Pour the mixture into the skillet and cook for an additional 3-5 minutes, until the sauce slightly thickens and coats the rolls.

11. Take the pan off the heat and serve garnished with a squeeze of fresh lime juice and green onions.

12. Serve and enjoy.

Plant-Based Seafood-Style Casserole

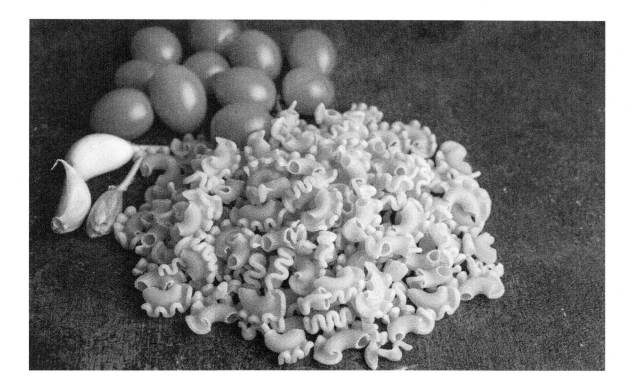

Veggies, pasta, and beans come together in a wholesome seafood-free, plant-based casserole to provide a wholesome weeknight meal.

Servings: 8

Total Time: 1hour 30mins

Ingredients:

Filling:

- 2 (14½ ounce) cans garbanzo beans (drained, 1 cup of liquid reserved)*
- 3 cups macaroni noodles
- 2 cups onion (peeled and diced)
- 8 medium Cremini mushrooms (sliced)
- 2 cups fresh green peas
- 1 medium tomato (thinly sliced)

Sauce:

- 3 cups plant milk
- 1 cup canned garbanzo bean liquid
- 2 tbsp soy sauce
- 1 tbsp kelp powder
- 1 tsp onion powder
- 2 tsp dry mustard powder
- 2 tbsp prepared mild mustard
- ½ tsp freshly ground black pepper

Directions:

1. Add the drained garbanzo beans to a bowl and mash with a fork, leaving a small number of the garbanzo beans whole. Set aside for a moment.

2. Next, prepare the sauce. In a bowl, combine the plant milk with the garbanzo bean liquid, soy sauce, kelp powder, onion powder, mustard powder, mild mustard, and black pepper. Stir and put to one side.

3. Preheat the main oven to 375 degrees F.

4. Bring a large pot of salted water to boil. Add the noodles and cook until al dente.

5. In the meantime, prepare the filling: Over moderate heat, heat a skillet. Add the onions and cook for 5 minutes, until softened. One tablespoon at a time, add water, to prevent them sticking.

6. Next, add the mushroom and stir to combine.

7. Stir in the peas followed by the garbanzo beans from Step 1 and mix thoroughly to combine.

8. Stir the sauce and add it to the skillet, mixing to combine.

9. Drain the pasta and add it to the skillet.

10. Transfer the ingredients from the skillet into a 9x13" casserole dish.

11. Arrange slices of tomato onto of the ingredients, and uncovered, bake in the preheated oven for 35-40 minutes, or until the top gently browns.

"Tuna" Mayo Stuffed Avocadoes

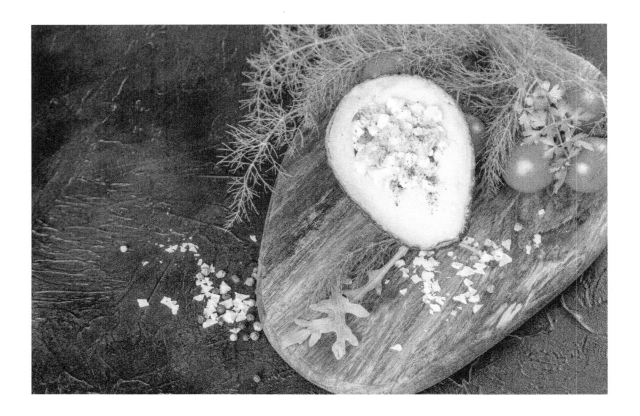

A nutritious and delicious lunchtime meal like these "tuna" mayo stuffed avocadoes will help you power through the rest of the day.

Servings: 2

Total Time: 10mins

Ingredients:

- 3 cups cooked white beans
- ½ cup yellow onion (finely chopped)
- 2 celery stalks (diced)
- 2 tsp dulse powder
- ½ tsp sea salt
- 1 tsp dried dill
- ¾ cup mayonnaise
- 2 ripe avocadoes (halved, destoned)

Directions:

1. Add the white beans to a food processor and pulse until chunky and chopped. Transfer to a bowl along with the onion, celery, dulse powder, sea salt, dried dill, and mayonnaise. Stir to combine.

2. Spoon the "tuna" mayo mixture evenly into the avocado halves and serve straight away.

Vegan Style 'Seafood' Cocktail

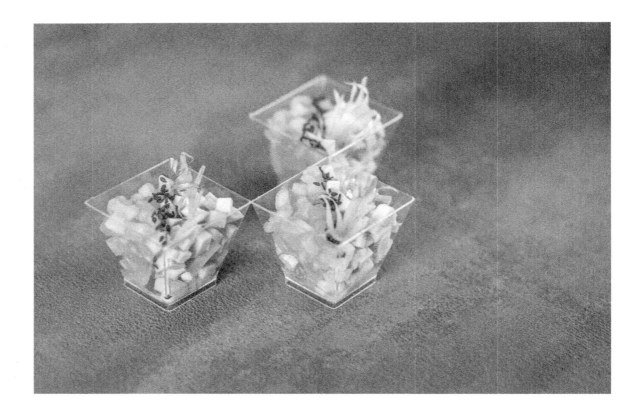

If you want to replicate crab in a seafood cocktail, then jackfruit is a great choice. Its tropical sweet flavor lends itself perfectly to this tasty appetizer to serve with tortilla chips.

Servings: 4

Total Time: 15mins

Ingredients:

- 1 (17 ounce) can green jackfruit in water
- ¼ tsp kelp powder
- ¼ tsp Old Bay Seasoning
- 2 Roma tomatoes (diced)
- 1 large avocado (peeled, pitted, and diced)
- ¼ cup organic ketchup
- ¼ cup white onion (peeled and diced)
- ¼ cup fresh cilantro leaves
- ½ jalapeño (seeded and stemmed)
- 1 tbsp fresh lemon juice
- ¼ tsp prepared, store-bought horseradish
- Tortilla chips (to serve)

Directions:

1. First, rinse the jackfruit, remove their seeds and with clean hands, gently squeeze out any excess water. Slice any hard chunks off from the ends and discard.

2. Using two metal forks shred the remaining jackfruit.

3. Add the jackfruits to a bowl and sprinkle kelp powder and Old Bay seasoning over the top. Mix thoroughly to combine. You can do this with your hands.

4. Add the tomatoes, avocado, ketchup, onion, cilantro, jalapeno, fresh lemon juice, and horseradish.

5. Transfer to the fridge to chill.

6. Serve with tortilla chips.

Watermelon Sashimi

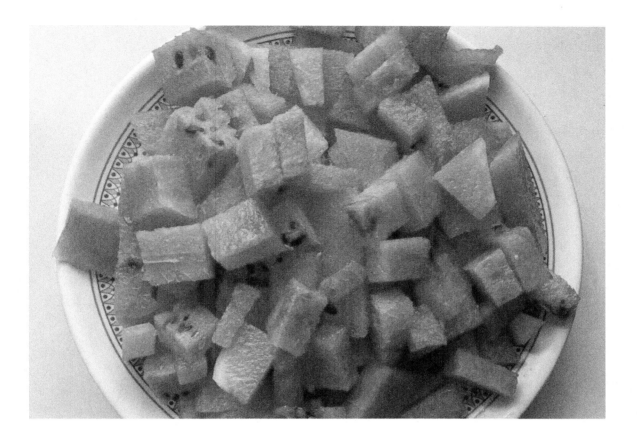

This watermelon sashimi dish is packed with flavor – it is the perfect light appetizer to enjoy during those hot summer months.

Servings: 4-6

Total Time: 10mins

Ingredients:

- 1 small watermelon (cut into triangles)
- 1 tbsp sesame oil
- 2½ tbsp tamari
- ¼ tsp wasabi
- 2 tbsp avocado (finely sliced)
- 2 tbsp pickled ginger
- ½ red onion (peeled, sliced thinly)
- 1½ tsp sesame seeds

Directions:

1. Pat the watermelon triangles with kitchen paper to absorb some of the excess juice.

2. Add the sesame oil, tamari, and wasabi to a small bowl and whisk to combine.

3. Transfer the watermelon to a serving platter and brush evenly with the prepared glaze.

4. Top each piece of watermelon with an equal amount of avocado, pickled ginger, and red onion.

5. Sprinkle over the sesame seeds.

6. Serve straight away!

Watermelon Poke Bowls

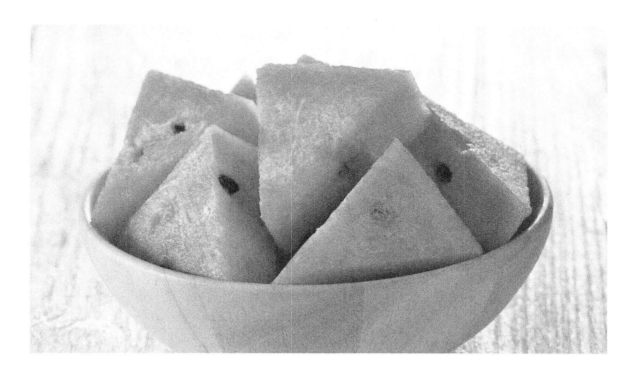

Poke is a native Hawaiian dish and typically consists of raw fish such as yellowfin tuna. You can still enjoy this Island delicacy while following a seafood-free diet, thanks to fresh and juicy watermelon.

Servings: 4

Total Time: 3hours 30mins

Ingredients:

Marinade:

- 2 tbsp toasted sesame oil
- 2 tbsp lime juice
- 2 tbsp rice vinegar
- 1 tbsp agave syrup
- 1 tsp lime zest
- 1 tbsp peanut butter
- 1 tbsp soy sauce
- 2 tbsp fresh ginger (grated)

Poke Bowl:

- 4 cups seedless watermelon (cubed)
- 1 cup dried black rice
- ¼ cup green onions (sliced thinly)
- 1 avocado (peeled, destoned, cubed)
- Toasted sesame seeds (to garnish)

Directions:

1. First, prepare the marinade. Add the sesame oil, lime juice, vinegar, agave syrup, lime zest, peanut butter, soy sauce, and ginger to a bowl and whisk to combine.

2. Add the watermelon cubes to a large ziplock bowl and pour in the marinade—seal and chill for 2 hours.

3. Place a skillet over moderate heat. Take the watermelon out of the marinade, do not discard the marinade.

4. Add the watermelon to the skillet and sauté for 4-5 minutes, stirring often.

5. Pour the marinade into the skillet and cook for 2-3 more minutes until thickened.

6. Transfer the contents of the skillet to a bowl and chill for half an hour.

7. Cook the rice using packet instructions.

8. Divide the cooked rice between 4 serving bowls and top each with an equal amount of watermelon, green onion, and avocado.

9. Garnish with sesame seeds and serve.

Author's Afterthoughts

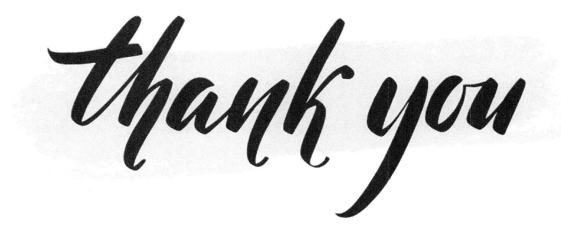

I would like to express my deepest thanks to you, the reader, for making this investment in one my books. I cherish the thought of bringing the love of cooking into your home.

With so much choice out there, I am grateful you decided to Purch this book and read it from beginning to end.

Please let me know by submitting an Amazon review if you enjoyed this book and found it contained valuable information to help you in your culinary endeavors. Please take a few minutes to express your opinion freely and honestly. This will help others make an informed decision on purchasing and provide me with valuable feedback.

Thank you for taking the time to review!

Christina Tosch

About the Author

Christina Tosch is a successful chef and renowned cookbook author from Long Grove, Illinois. She majored in Liberal Arts at Trinity International University and decided to pursue her passion of cooking when she applied to the world renowned Le Cordon Bleu culinary school in Paris, France. The school was lucky to recognize the immense talent of this chef and she excelled in her courses, particularly Haute Cuisine. This skill was recognized and rewarded by several highly regarded Chicago restaurants, where she was offered the prestigious position of head chef.

Christina and her family live in a spacious home in the Chicago area and she loves to grow her own vegetables and herbs in the garden she lovingly cultivates on her sprawling estate. Her and her husband have two beautiful children, 3 cats, 2 dogs and a parakeet they call Jasper. When Christina is not hard at work creating beautiful meals for Chicago's elite, she is hard at work writing engaging e-books of which she has sold over 1500.

Make sure to keep an eye out for her latest books that offer helpful tips, clear instructions and witty anecdotes that will bring a smile to your face as you read!

Printed in Great Britain
by Amazon